MOVING ANALYTICS

THRIVING WITH HEART FAILURE

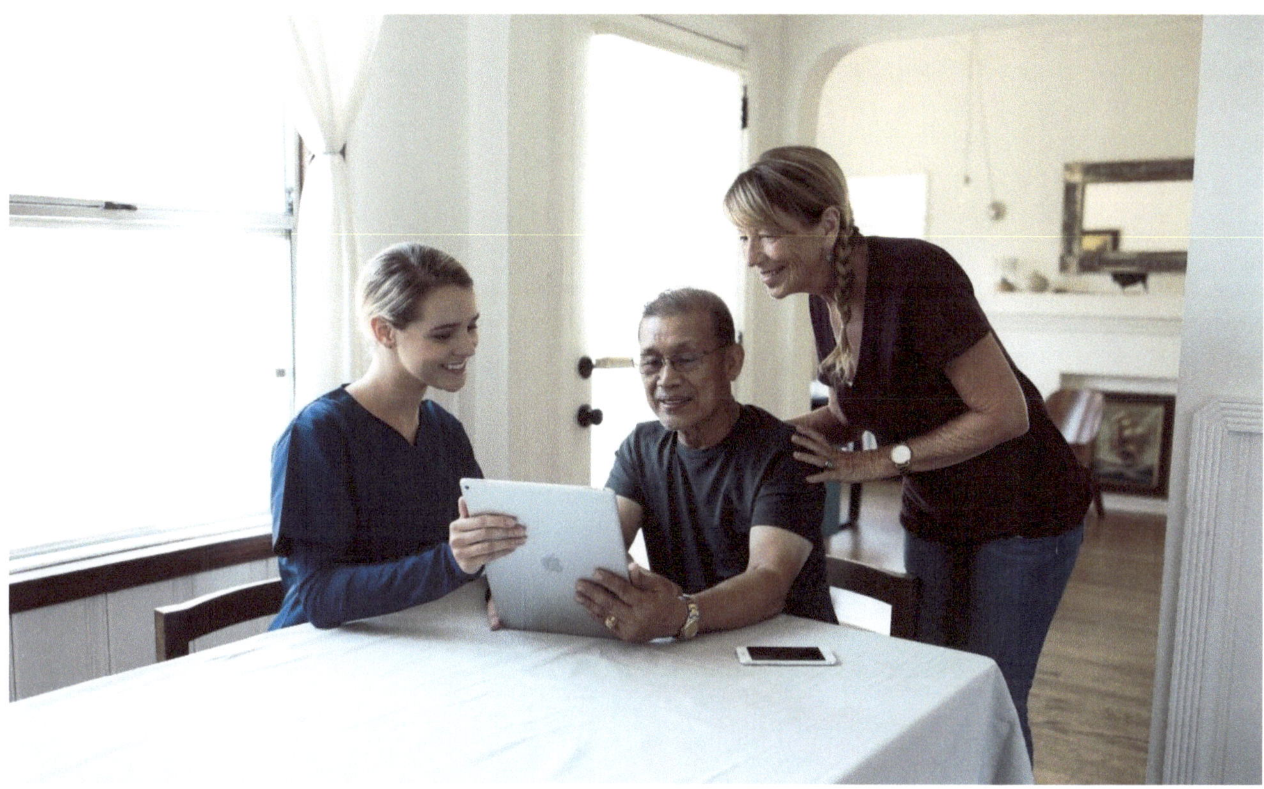

INTRODUCTION

What is heart failure?

Heart failure, also called congestive heart failure, can occur when the heart loses some of its pumping power. The heart still beats, but not as well as before, so it has to work harder to do its job. Heart failure can be mild, moderate or severe. It is a chronic condition, which means that it does not go away.

What causes heart failure?

Heart disease may result from:
- Coronary artery disease
- A past heart attack (myocardial infarction)
- High blood pressure (hypertension)
- Heart valve disease (valve stenosis or insufficiency)
- Heart muscle problems (cardiomyopathy)
- Congenital (born with) heart disease
- Infection of the heart valves or muscle
- Toxins (e.g. Drugs, alcohol, chemotherapy)
- Other medical conditions (thyroid problems, diabetes etc.)

Over time, these conditions decrease the heart's pumping power. You should ask your doctor or nurse what caused your heart failure.

How does the heart work?

The human heart is about the size of a fist. It has four chambers that squeeze and relax with each heartbeat. Four valves control the flow of blood between the chambers and out to the lungs and the body. Blood carries oxygen and nutrients through the blood vessels (arteries) to your organs (brain, kidneys, etc.) and tissues (muscles and skin).

Blood returns to the heart through the veins. The heart then pumps the blood to the lungs to get fresh oxygen and nutrients that are brought back to the heart. Then the process starts over again.

When you sit still, your body's need for oxygen and nutrients is low. The heart pumps just fast enough to meet these needs. When you are active or under mental stress, the heart must work harder to meet the body's increased needs. The heart beats faster and the blood vessels expand to be sure that all the parts of the body get enough oxygen and nutrients.

What are the effects of heart failure?

In heart failure, the heart does not pump blood through the body as well as it should. Three problems may result:

1. Blood may back up into the veins. This backup forces fluid into the tissues causing swelling. Usually the ankles, feet and legs swell. Sometimes the abdomen (belly) and liver swell also.
2. When the left side of the heart does not pump properly, fluid may build up in the lungs. This condition is called "pulmonary edema" and causes patients to feel very short of breath and tired.
3. Less blood reaches the tissues and organs, so they do not get as much food and oxygen as they may need. Patients may feel very tired as a result.

What are the symptoms of heart failure?

The most common symptom of heart failure is shortness of breath. It may occur with your usual activity, during exercise, or when you lie down. You may even wake up at night feeling short of breath.

Other symptoms include fatigue, (feeling tired), swelling in your legs, ankles or abdomen (belly), sudden weight gain, a dry cough, fainting, feeling dizzy or irregular heartbeats. You should know how to respond to a change in symptoms. The section in this workbook called "Monitoring Your Symptoms" can help you.

How is heart failure managed?

You play a key role in managing your heart failure. Your doctor will prescribe medicines and a low-sodium diet to help treat your symptoms. However, you must help with the day-to-day management of the disease. Here's what you should know:

Medicines

The most common medicines for heart failure are water pills (diuretics), a drug to lower heart rate and blood pressure (beta-blockers) and drugs which make it easier for the heart to pump (ACE inhibitors). Because you must take so many medicines, you should know the name of each drug, when the best time is for you to take your drugs, and whether there are side effects that you should report to your doctor or nurse. Your nurse will help you develop a system to remind you to take your medicines.

Diet

You must limit the amount of sodium you eat. Sodium, which comes from salt, causes your body to hold fluid. The extra fluid puts more strain on your heart. You should learn which foods have a lot of sodium or salt so you can avoid them. You should also limit the amount of alcohol you drink and lose weight if you are overweight. You will receive guidelines to help you make these changes in your eating habits.

Activity and Exercise

You may need to limit some activities if your heart failure is severe. Talk to your doctor or nurse about how you feel when you do certain activities. You may be able to be more active if your medicine is changed or a dose is increased. A regular exercise program often helps patients feel better. Be sure to check with your nurse or doctor for the right exercise program.

Daily Weights

You should weigh yourself every morning right after you get out of bed and urinate. A 2.5 lb. weight gain in 1 day, or even a 5 lb. weight gain over 5 days, may mean that your body is holding extra fluid. If you notice such a weight gain, report it to your doctor or nurse right away. Make sure you have a good scale to weigh yourself daily.

Reporting symptoms

If you have a symptom that gets worse, you should report it right away. You should also report any side effects from your medicines. Do not wait until your next doctor's visit to report symptoms or side effects. A change in symptoms may mean that your heart failure is getting worse or that a medicine needs to be changed. Always check with your doctor or nurse if you are not sure about a symptom or side effect.

Looking to the future

Living with heart failure means changing your lifestyle. However, if you follow the recommendations in this booklet and become an active partner in your care, your quality of life will be improved. Your doctor, nurse, family and friends can help you.

MONITORING YOUR SYMPTOMS

Heart failure makes it harder for the heart to work properly. Two main problems result:

1. Fluid can back up in the lungs, legs and other parts of the body, which causes shortness of breath and/or swelling.
2. Not enough blood reaches the organs and muscles, causing you to feel tired and/or short of breath.

Even if you are taking medicines, eating a low-sodium diet and exercising, you may still have symptoms. Your nurse will ask you about your symptoms. We ask that you rate your symptoms from mild to severe. Also, think about the questions listed below related to your symptoms.

Do you have shortness of breath during exercise or at rest?
- Does it wake you up at night?
- Does it come on when you lie down and go away when you sit up?

Do you have swelling or bloating of your abdomen (belly)?
- Is there swelling in your legs or ankles, especially at the end of the day?
- Have you gained 2.5 lbs. in a day? Or, have you gained 5 lbs. in 5 days?

Have you had any chest discomfort? If so, what does it feel like? (pressure, tightness, burning, aching, etc.)
- Does it move? (down your arm, into your jaw or back, etc.)
- Does it wake you up at night?

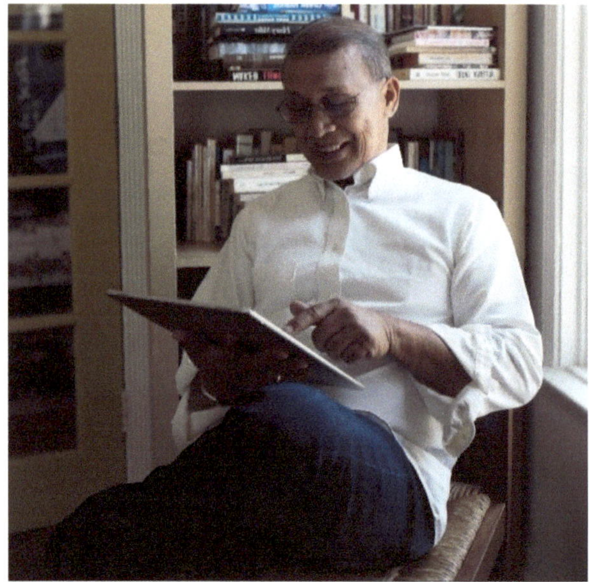

- Does it occur with exercise or other activities?

Other important symptoms to monitor include:
- Lack of energy; feeling tired
- Cough
- Fainting
- Loss of appetite
- Irregular heart beats
- Slow or fast pulse
- Feeling dizzy upon standing up
- Increased urination at night

Call your doctor or nurse if you notice new or worsening symptoms.

MANAGING HEART FAILURE: WHEN TO SEEK HELP

If you want to feel better and stay out of the hospital, getting answers to your medical questions right away can help in many cases.

You need to know about three areas in order to take good care of yourself:
- What signs and symptoms (how you feel) are important?
- When should I call someone? Now or later?
- Whom should I call?

The information below will help you to know which symptoms require prompt action, and to make an action plan for reaching the right health care professional.

What symptoms need to be reported?

People with heart failure often feel tired or have some shortness of breath or swelling of their feet, ankles or abdomen (belly) due to excess water. Many people have also had a heart attack and continue to have chest discomfort due to coronary heart disease. The two most common symptoms that require you act right away are shortness of breath and chest discomfort.

Shortness of breath:

You should call your nurse or doctor during the hours of _____-______ at this number (___) ___-_____ for shortness of breath that changes from mild to moderate during your daytime activities, appears at night, especially when you lie in bed, or increases over a 24-hour period. An increase in your diuretic (water pill) prescribed by your doctor may be enough to control your condition and avoid a visit to the emergency room.

NOTE: For shortness of breath that becomes severe in 12 hours or less, especially at night, you should call 911 or go to the emergency room.

Chest Discomfort:

Discomfort under your breastbone (pressure, tightness, burning or squeezing), that is new for you or that worsens also requires you to act right away.

- If you have chest discomfort under your breastbone that comes on at rest or lasts more than 2 minutes after you stop physical activity and you do not have nitroglycerin, call 911 or go to the nearest emergency room.
- If you have nitroglycerine, take one tablet or spray dose. If after 5 minutes the chest pain is not better or gets worse, **call 911 or other emergency services immediately**.

What symptoms require immediate action?

Some symptoms require immediate action. This means calling 911 or going directly to the emergency room. These include:
- <u>Severe shortness of breath,</u> especially if it awakens you from sleep.
- <u>Chest discomfort</u> that does not go away after 5 minutes with nitroglycerin or which occurs with nausea, vomiting, or discomfort radiating to your arm or jaw.
- <u>Severe dizziness or lightheadedness</u> that lasts 10 minutes or longer or fainting.

Most symptoms don't occur suddenly. Prompt action on your part may help to prevent more serious problems and may even prevent a visit to the emergency room or hospital.

- <u>Fast</u> or <u>irregular heartbeat</u>, especially when accompanied by shortness of breath, chest discomfort or dizziness.
- <u>Swelling of your face</u>, <u>lips or mouth</u> or difficulty swallowing or breathing after starting a new medicine.
- <u>Signs of a possible stroke</u>, including: the worst headache you've ever had, sudden dramatic change in vision, sudden weakness in the arm, hand or leg, numbness on one side of your face or body, or having a hard time talking or understanding what others are saying.
- <u>If you are taking Warfarin</u>, a blood-thinning medication, you should go to the emergency room if you have any black or bloody stools, coughing up blood or vomit bloody or coffee grounds material or if you notice bloody urine.
- Increased urination at night

What about other symptoms?

Most of the other symptoms that you are likely to have can be handled during the day by calling your nurse. Don't forget to leave a message even if you aren't sure about a new symptom or a change in a usual symptom.

Whom do I contact after hours?

Most symptoms develop slowly, not rapidly. Symptoms often increase gradually over many hours or days. The sooner you call for help the less anxious you will feel and the better your problem can be managed.

Below are the recommendations for whom you should call about your condition at any time:

- For severe symptoms or symptoms that become much worse over 12 hours, call 911 or go to the nearest emergency room.
- For changes in your symptoms over a 12-24-hour period, for routine questions, or when a situation is not urgent your nurse or doctor.
- If you are unsure whether your symptom is serious, and you can't reach your nurse, call your doctor's office (___) ___-_____.

Your nurse may arrange for a doctor visit, an urgent care appointment, or a phone call with your doctor.

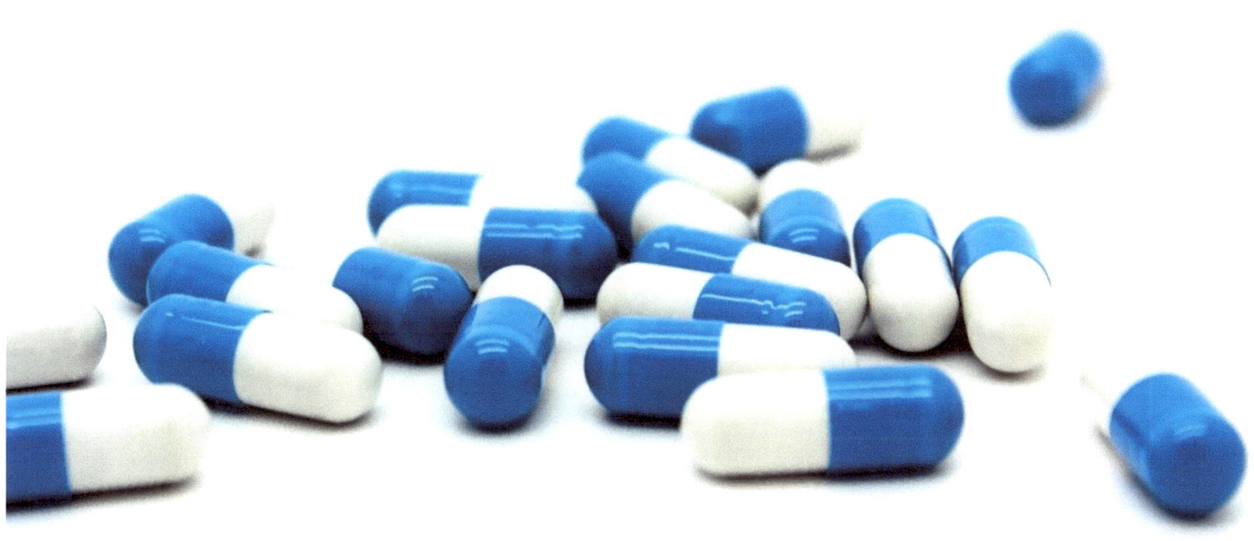

MEDICINES AND HEART FAILURE

There are now many medicines used to help the heart pump more and become stronger. Some of these medicines are used to decrease symptoms. Others help to prevent heart failure from getting worse. This section below will highlight the classes of medicines most often used to treat heart failure prescribed by healthcare professionals. They are listed here in alphabetical order but not in order of importance.

Angiotensin Converting Enzyme Inhibitors (ACE Inhibitors)

ACE Inhibitors act by decreasing how hard the heart must work. They prevent the body from producing angiotensin, which can cause blood vessels to tighten and raise blood pressure. By causing the blood vessels in the body to dilate (open), blood pressure goes down and the heart doesn't have to work as hard. ACE inhibitors not only take the workload off the heart but also have a positive effect on the kidney. If taken regularly they can decrease the chances of dying and decrease symptoms.

Side effects will be less if ACE inhibitors are started at a low dose and gradually increased. The most common side effect of an ACE inhibitor is feeling dizzy or lightheaded, a slight skin rash or having a dry cough. Because ACE inhibitors can lower blood pressure, the first dose may be given when lying down or at night. The dose can then be changed in a few days as needed. If you take an ACE inhibitor, your doctor will likely ask you to get a potassium blood test as these medicines can sometimes increase the potassium level in the blood causing irregular heartbeats. You will also be asked to get a lab test for your kidney function and potassium level. If you have any light-headedness, cough, rash or swelling of your face (which is rare), you should contact your doctor immediately.

Listed below are the most common ACE Inhibitors.

GENERIC NAME	TRADE NAME
Captopril	(Capoten)
Enalapril	(Vasotec)
Fosinopril	(Monopril)
Lisinopril	(Prinivil, Zestril)
Perindopril	(Aceon)
Quinapril	(Acupril)
Ramipril	(Altace)
Trandolapril	(Mavik)
Benazepril	(Lotensin)
Moexipril	(Univasc)

Angiotensin Receptor Blockers (ARB's)

If you can't take an ace inhibitor, (ACE), you will likely be asked to take a medicine to lower blood pressure known as an ARB. ARB's have almost the same effect for heart failure patients as ACE inhibitors and prevent the body from using a substance called angiotensin. Thus, they lower blood pressure and take the workload off the heart. Like the ACE inhibitors, you will be asked to get lab tests so your doctor can observe your kidney function and a potassium level to make sure it is not out of range. These medicines can also cause you to feel dizzy or lightheaded. Other possible side effects include rash, swelling of the face or kidney problems. As with ACE Inhibitors, if you have any allergic reaction to an ARB it should be reported to your doctor.

GENERIC NAME	TRADE NAME
Candesartan	(Atacand)
Losartan	(Cozaar)
Valsartan	(Diovan)
Irbesartan	(Avapro)
Eprosartan	(Teventen)
Telmisartan	(Micardis)

Beta blockers

These medicines have been used in heart patients for over 40 years. When the heart does not pump as well, certain hormones increase to try and balance decreased heart function. The hormone, adrenaline, binds to the heart muscle and causes the heart to beat harder and faster which over time can weaken the heart. Beta-blockers lower the heart rate and blood pressure by blocking adrenaline. A few beta-blockers such as carvedilol (Coreg), sustained-release metoprolol (Toprol XL) and bisoprolol (Zebeta) have not only improved symptoms but also survival in those with heart failure.

GENERIC NAME	TRADE NAME
Captopril	(Capoten)
Enalapril	(Vasotec)
Fosinopril	(Monpril)
Lisinopril	(Prinivil,Zestril)
Perindpril	(Aceon)
Quinapril	(Acupril)
Ramipril	(Altace)
Trandolapril	(Mavik)
Benazepril	(Lotensin)
Moexipril	(Univasc)

The most common side effects of beta-blockers include feeling tired, weak or dizzy and a decrease in sexual function and slowing of the heart rate. Severe symptoms of feeling light-headed, fainting, or breathing difficulties are less common but are also possible side effects. Be sure to call your doctor if you have a severe side effect.

GENERIC NAME	TRADE NAME
Bisoprolol	(Zebeta)
Metoprolol Succinate	(Toprol XL)
Carvedilol	(Coreg)
Carvedilol CR	(Coreg CR)
Acebutolol	(Sectral)
Atenolol	(Tenormin)
Betaxolol	(Kerlone)
Labetolol	(Trandate)
Nadolol	(Corgard)
Penbutolol	(Levatol)
Pindolol	(Visken)
Propranolol	(Inderal)
Timolol	(Blocadren)

Digitalis

This medicine, has been shown to decrease symptoms and readmission to the hospital by helping the heart to pump better. It is also used to slow the heart rate and improve irregular heartbeats. If you have previously been in the hospital for heart failure you may be asked to start Digitalis. Side effects include loss of appetite, nausea, vomiting and in some cases headaches. More severe side effects that must be reported to your doctor immediately include vision problems such as seeing blue, yellow or green colors or having blurred vision.

GENERIC NAME	TRADE NAME
Digoxin	(Digitek, Lanoxin, Lanoxicaps)
Digitoxin	(Crystodigin)

Diuretics (water pills)

Diuretics, or water pills, are used to relieve the fluid-build up that may occur when the heart does not function as well as it should. Water pills relieve the fluid that often builds up in the legs or abdomen. At times, two different diuretics may be used to help with heart failure: one to lower blood pressure and the other to remove fluid. Special diuretics such as spironolactone often work in combination with other diuretics to get rid of fluid. Spironolactone blocks a chemical called aldosterone, which causes the body to hold in fluid and water. This pill has been shown to not only relieve symptoms but also improve survival.

Side effects from diuretics may include needing to urinate frequently and slight dizziness. More severe side effects include low blood pressure, poor kidney function and low or high potassium levels. Spironolactone has been known to cause high blood potassium levels and you may be asked to get a lab test after starting this medicine.

GENERIC NAME	TRADE NAME
Furosemide	(Lasix)
Bumetanide	(Bumex)
Eplerenone	(Inspra)
Hydrochlorothiazide	(Hydrodiuril)
Spironolactone	(Aldactone)
Torsemide	(Demadex)
Metolazone	(Zaroxolyn)
Chlorothiazide	(Diuril)

Vasodilators

If needed, this class of medicines may do many things. For example, nitroglycerin relieves chest discomfort associated with heart disease. Vasodilators are also used to relieve fluid retention (buildup) for people who have heart failure. These medicines open up blood vessels allowing more blood and oxygen to get to the heart. Possible side effects can include feeling dizzy or lightheaded when changing positions, headaches, feeling flushed or redness of the face, and nasal congestion. In some cases, Hydralazine may also cause joint pain.

GENERIC NAME	TRADE NAME
Hydralazine	(Apresoline)
Isosorbide dinitrate	(Isordil)
Isosorbide mononitrate	(Imdur or Ismo)
Nitroglycerin Patch	(Nitrodur or Minitran)

Other medicines to treat heart failure

While not listed here you may be also asked to take a few other medicines if needed to help with heart failure. These may include a potassium supplement if you take a diuretic that depletes potassium, a blood thinner if you develop blood clots in your legs or another part of the body, or an anti-arrhythmic medicine to treat an irregular heart rhythm such as atrial fibrillation. Be sure to go over all of the important information about taking any of these medicines with your doctor or nurse.

Newest agents in the treatment of heart failure

Two new medicines have recently been released to help people with heart failure. The first medicine (Entresol) a combination neprilysin inhibitor and ARB. Neprilysin is a peptide that causes vasoconstriction (narrowing) and fluid retention (build-up). When a neprilysin inhibitor is paired with the ARB, valsartan, the combination reduces hospitalizations and improve survival. It is given twice per day in low doses of both medicines and is gradually increased. Severe side effects may include swelling of the face, lips, tongue and throat. If these symptoms occur, seeking medical help immediately is important. These medicines are given if people are not taking a regular ACE inhibitor or ARB.

Another new medicine is Ivabradine (Corlanor) that is used to help reduce readmissions to the hospital. It works on the conduction system of the heart and results in a decrease in heart rate. The most common side effects of Ivabradine are blurred vision, feeling dizzy, fast or irregular heartbeat, headache or shortness of breath. It may also cause atrial fibrillation, which is a fast-irregular heart rhythm that needs to be reported to your doctor. Ivabradine is most often taken twice per day with food.

GENERIC NAME	TRADE NAME
Calcium Channel Blocker/Inhibitor	
Ivabradine	(Corlanor)
Angiotensin Receptor Neprilysin Inhibitors (ARNIs)	
Sacubitril/ Valsartan	(Ernesto)

Over-the-counter medicines

Your heart failure medicines are needed to prevent further heart weakness and to relieve your symptoms. Some medicines that you purchase may interfere with your prescribed medicines. Before you take any decongestant or antihistamine for a cold or allergy, talk with your doctor or nurse. You should **avoid** taking decongestants. You should also tell them if you are taking an acid blocker to relieve stomach upset. If you take an anti-inflammatory medicine for pain, you should also inform your doctor or nurse. And always remember that your medicine list should not only include your prescribed medicines but also any supplements or herbals you are taking.

Below are some facts about the medicines that might interfere with your heart failure medicines.

Decongestants and antihistamines

Decongestants reduce swelling or congestion in the nasal passages but can also make your heart work harder. You need to **avoid** taking decongestants. Most of the medicines used to treat a cold or flu contain decongestants.

Antihistamines are most often used to treat allergies or hay fever. Because they don't constrict (narrow) vessels in the nasal passages, they are safer than decongestants. But it is best to pick the right ones. Avoid taking a medicine with pseudoephedrine. Instead take a safer medicine like diphenhydramine such as Benadryl. And remember, do not take antihistamines combined with decongestants like Sudafed. Your pharmacist can help you find the best antihistamine.

Non-steroidal anti-inflammatories

Non-steroidal anti-inflammatory medicines are often used for joint or muscle pain. But for patients with heart failure they can cause fluid buildup and kidney problems. It is much safer to stay away from these medicines such as Ibuprofen (Advil, Motrin or Nuprin), Naprosyn (Aleve), and Celecoxib (Celebrex—often used for arthritis). Choose to use Tylenol (Acetaminophen) for pain relief.

Acid blocker

Acid blockers reduce acid in the stomach. Indigestion or heartburn is often caused by this build-up of acid, but some medicines can interfere with your heart failure medicines. Choose antacids such as ranitidine HCL (zantac), famotidine (Pepcid) or nizatidine (Axid), instead of cimetidine (Tagamet).

Talk to your pharmacist or doctor about which medicines you might take.

Tips for taking your medicines

Please take your medicines. Taken in proper doses, medicines can allow you to be more active, icrease your exercise ability and most certainly they will decrease your symptoms. Many studies show your medicines can prevent visits to the emergency room and being admitted to the hospital. Forgetting medicines is likely to cause increased shortness of breath and weight gain.

Taking medicines isn't easy. Almost 50% of all people do not take their medicines correctly. They miss a dose, take a medicine at the wrong time, take an incorrect dose, or fail to have a prescription filled. When there are many medicines to keep track of, it becomes even harder.

- ☐ Do you ever forget to take your medications?
- ☐ Are you careless at times about taking your medications?
- ☐ When you feel better, do you sometimes stop taking your medicine?
- ☐ Sometimes if you feel worse when you take your medicine, do you stop taking it?

If you responded "yes" to any of the above questions, here are some tips to help you:

If you sometimes forget…

- Use a pillbox for your medicines.
- Buy an inexpensive watch that you can set to remind you of every dose.
- Ask a family member to help you remember to take your pills.
- Post signs on the refrigerator, bathroom mirror or near the TV to help you.

If you are careless at times…

- Record when you have taken your medicine.
- If timing is a problem, take your medicine during a daily routine such as when you wake up, brush your teeth, or with meals.
- Ask a family member to give you your medicine when it is time to take it.

If you feel better and you sometimes stop taking your medicines…

Decide why. Are you having side effects? Do your medicines cost too much? Is taking them a hassle?
Talk to your doctor or nurse about what can be done to make it easier for you.
- Keep in mind that these medicines are **helping** you feel better. If you stop taking them, your illness may get worse.

If you feel worse when you take your medicine and you stop them…

Are you having side effects? If so, **talk to your doctor or nurse.** There may be ways to improve the side effects, or you may need your medicine changed.

A few more tips…

Know the name, **dose**, and **reason** you are taking each medicine. Carry a list of your medicines always.

- Plan a week in advance to have your medicines refilled…mark it on the calendar as a reminder.
- If cost is an issue, ask your doctor or pharmacist about a less expensive medicine.

Plan. If your daily schedule is disrupted by plans for a vacation or other events, write notes to yourself and place them in places where you are sure to see them. Pocket calendars may also be helpful. If you need more reminders and greater support from family and friends, be sure to tell them.
Taking medication is not easy. Be sure to talk to your family, nurse or doctor if you have problems or concerns with your medicine.

ACTIVITY AND EXERCISE

Heart failure patients differ in the amount of activity they can do. Some people must limit their daily activities, while others are able to continue doing everything. You will likely need to pace yourself and allow time for rest between activities. Read this section carefully; learn the guidelines for activity and exercise. Your nurse will discuss personal limits with you.

You can expect to have good days and bad days. You **must** note how you feel. If you don't feel well or have a fever, you should skip most activities. Just rest at home that day.

Know the symptoms and signs that you should report to your nurse or doctor.

You should wait at least one hour after eating to exercise or do an activity (such as bathing or household chores). It is okay to be active before you eat.

Tips for everyday activities

Limit baths or showers to 10 minutes or less. Use warm water-- **never** hot, steamy water.

Save your energy by sitting down while you dry off, get dressed, shave or comb your hair. If you need to, prop your elbows on a table to shave, put on makeup or comb your hair.

Give yourself breaks between your daily care activities. Allow 10 to 20 minutes between bathing, dressing or shaving.

Tips for household chores

Ask for help with household chores if you need it or hire someone to do the chores for you.

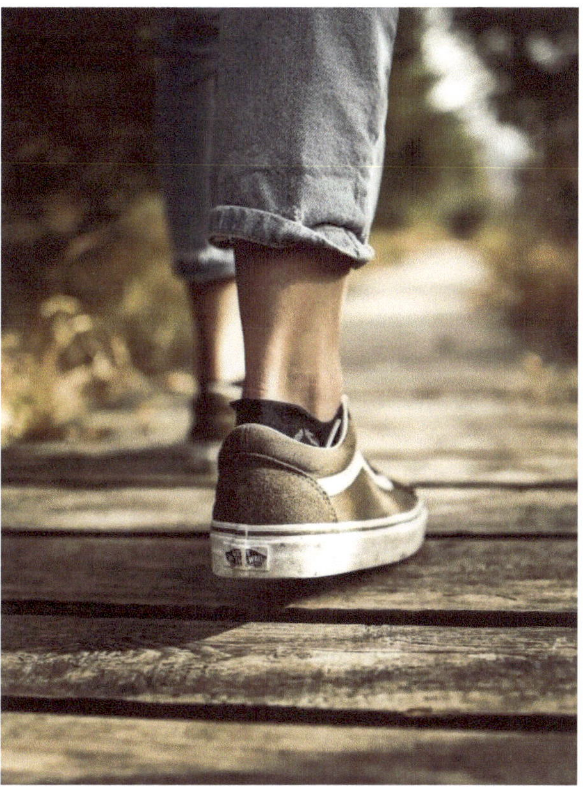

Space out your tasks (errands, cooking, cleaning, etc.). Take time to rest in between.

Using your arms for a long period of time makes the heart work extra hard. Therefore, activities such as sweeping, vacuuming and raking leaves will make you tire easily. Break these actions into parts and rest in-between. For example, mow one strip of lawn, sit and enjoy the fresh air, then mow another strip.

Don't lift or push more than **5** pounds at a time. Be careful when moving wet laundry, pulling up a mattress to change sheets, ironing, taking out the garbage, etc.

Organize your home to help you save energy. For example, have a chair or stool to sit on when cutting vegetables; keep cooking supplies together within easy reach of the sink or stove; and keep cleaning supplies together where they are easy to use.

Use a wheeled cart to help you move things from room to room.

Sit down to iron and use more perm-pressed clothing.

Tips for leisure activities

Do something you like to do every day (window shopping, working at the computer, gardening, calling a friend, watching a movie, etc.).

Plan to rest before a party or special outing so you will have more energy.

Keep your legs elevated when sitting.

Do not kneel or squat for long periods (for instance, when gardening). Sit on a low chair instead.

Sexual activity

Don't be afraid to talk to your nurse if you have a question or have noticed a change related to sexual activity. Keep in mind that the energy required for sexual intercourse is about the same as climbing two flights of stairs.

Don't engage in sexual activity right after you eat. Mornings may be a good time because you are well rested.

If you tire easily, try to avoid putting full weight on your arms; try side-by-side or another comfortable position.

Hugging, kissing and handholding are ways to show love that use very little energy!

Daily exercise

Regular exercise may help you feel better mentally and give you more energy for other activities. An ideal exercise program includes 20 to 30 minutes of exercise every day. Most patients with heart failure choose to walk for exercise, although you may prefer to bicycle or swim.

Your nurse will help you work out a good exercise program. You may need to start very slowly, perhaps walking only a few minutes twice a day in your home. You should stretch your muscles before and after exercise to avoid injury, no matter how short or long your exercise time.

Your exercise routine is made up of three parts:
1. Warm up (stretching and movement to get the body ready for exercise)
2. Exercise
3. Cool down (stretching while the heart rate returns to resting level)

You should not do isometric exercises, weight lifting, competitive sports or contact sports unless these have been discussed with your doctor.

Tips for safe exercise

- Dress for the weather, but do not exercise in very hot or very cold weather.
- Be sure to warm up before exercise. Warm up may include starting your exercise at a slower pace and then stretching your muscles.
- You should expect to breathe a little harder and you may sweat while you exercise. You should be able to talk comfortably even if you are breathing harder.
- Another way to monitor shortness of breath during exercise is to rate

yourself on a scale of 1 to 4. Give yourself a "1" if you are mildly short of breath and a "4" if you are very short of breath. You will likely be somewhere in between. If you rate yourself a "3" or higher during exercise, slow down or stop exercising until you feel comfortable.

- It is easy to overdo exercise when you are at high altitudes or have not exercised for a few days due to illness. At these times, you should start your exercise at a low level and exercise for a shorter period than usual.
- Be sure to cool down after you exercise and before you shower.
- You may enjoy exercise more if you do it with a friend or family member.

Listen to your body

You should learn to "listen to your body" when exercising or performing other physical tasks. A scale that is often used to measure your level of intensity (how hard you work) during exercise is the "Borg Scale of Perceived Exertion" also known as the Rating of Perceived Exertion or RPE Scale. This scale offers a way for you to think about how hard you are working when you exercise. It also is a good way of telling your nurse how you are doing with your exercise program

You should not exercise above 14 on the scale. There may be days when you can work in the gray area (12-14) without any problems. Other days it may be harder. If you have new symptoms or your symptoms get worse while exercising or doing other activities, **tell your doctor or nurse** right away.

6		**6-8** levels are like sitting quietly.
7	**Very, very light**	
8		
9	**Very light**	**9-11** levels are more activity such as warm up and cool down stretches and movements.
10		
11	**Fairly light**	
12		**12-14** levels are activities where you can talk. In this range you may breathe a little harder and sweat.
13	**Somewhat hard**	
14		
15	**Hard**	**15-20** levels are **hard** and breathing becomes more difficult. If you are in this range, you need to **slow down - you are overdoing it!**
16		
17	**Very hard**	
18		
19	**Very, very hard**	
20		

From Borg, GA: Med Sci Sports Exer 14:377-387, 1982

Signs and symptoms with activity

You must stay alert to signs and symptoms when you are active. Watch for **chest discomfort, strong fast heart beats, severe shortness of breath, a lightheaded feeling or feeling dizzy.** If you notice any of these symptoms, slow down right away and find a place to sit and rest.

- If you have chest discomfort or pain that lasts more than 2 minutes after you stop physical activity and you do not have nitroglycerin, **call 911** or go to the nearest emergency room.
- If you have nitroglycerine, take one tablet or spray dose. If after 5 minutes the chest pain is not better

or gets worse, **call 911 or other emergency services immediately**.

If you are having strong fast heart beats, severe shortness of breath, are very light- headed or very dizzy for 10 minutes or longer, or if you have fainted, **call the paramedics (911) or go to the nearest emergency room.**

Call your nurse right away if your <u>usual</u> symptoms get worse. These include angina (chest discomfort), shortness of breath, cough, leg swelling, fatigue or bloating. You may need to slow down or cut back on your activity, or you may be building up fluid.

How to check your pulse

In this program you may be asked to check your pulse (heart rate) when you exercise. Use the following steps to practice counting your pulse at rest. Once you know how to check your pulse at rest, it will be much easier to check it during exercise.

1. Make sure that you can see a watch or clock that has a second hand. You may also use an Apple Watch or Fitbit to see your pulse.
2. If you are checking your pulse, use your first two fingers to find your pulse. You can find it either on the thumb side of your wrist or on one side your neck, one inch from your windpipe. If you have trouble finding your pulse, try using three fingers instead of two.
3. Count your pulse for ten seconds. The longer you count your pulse the more it drops. Therefore, you should only count it for ten seconds.
4. Now multiply your pulse by six to get your pulse rate per minute. This is your resting heart rate or pulse rate.

5. If you have a hard time finding your pulse, use a pen to make a small mark on your wrist that will help you find the right spot the next time you take your pulse rate.

How to get your pulse rate

Number of beats in 10 seconds   X   6   =   Pulse rate per/min

NOTE: If you have a pacemaker or atrial fibrillation, you should count your pulse by either:

1. Taking it for 30 seconds and multiplying by 2, or
2. Taking it for 60 seconds to get the pulse rate.

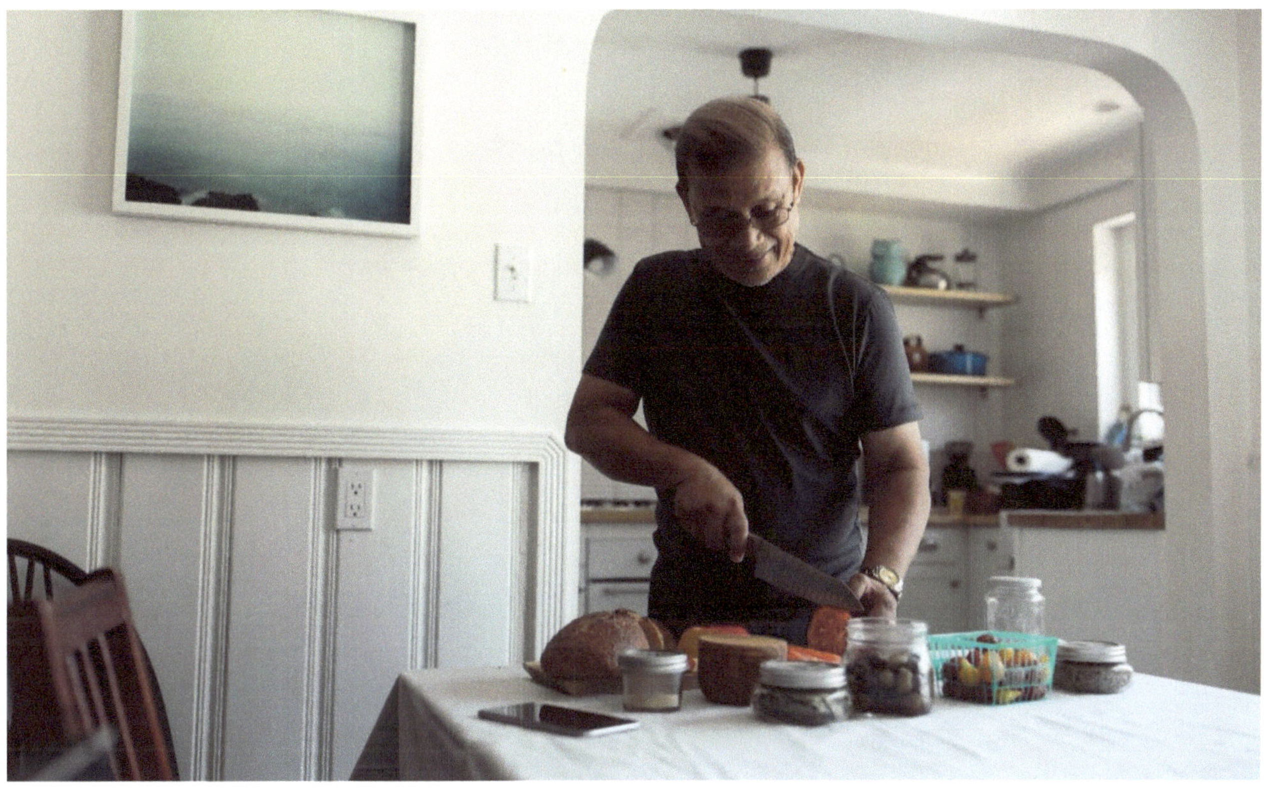

LIMITING DIETARY SODIUM

If you have heart failure, this chapter is very important for you. Limiting sodium and taking your medicines as prescribed are the keys to managing your condition.

If you have high blood pressure, limiting sodium may help bring your blood pressure down. However, this doesn't work for everyone. The only way to know if limiting sodium will help lower your blood pressure is to give it a try.

Test Yourself

Here is a quick test to find out if your diet is already low in sodium. Put a check by the things you do most of the time:

- ☐ I avoid adding salt during cooking and at the table.
- ☐ I use herbs and spices instead of salt to flavor foods.
- ☐ I rinse canned vegetables, chicken and fish before eating them.
- ☐ I read food labels for sodium content and sodium-containing ingredients.
- ☐ I eat processed foods (frozen meals, canned soups, luncheon meats) no more than twice a week.
- ☐ I rarely use salty condiments like mustard, soy sauce, barbecue sauce, olives or pickles.

How did you do?

- People with heart failure should have all items checked.
- People with high blood pressure should have at least four items checked.
- People with either condition should have at least three items checked.

- About half the sodium we eat comes from processed foods: snack foods, frozen foods, canned, pickled and smoked foods, and certain dairy foods like cheese and buttermilk.
- About one-third comes from the salt shaker during cooking or at the table. A teaspoon of salt contains 2000 mg. of sodium.
- A small amount of sodium comes from water and foods that naturally contain sodium, like meat, fish, milk and vegetables.
- Additional sodium comes from leavening agents (baking soda and baking powder) and flavorings like soy sauce, MSG, catsup, mustard and chili sauce.

RECOMMENDED SODIUM INTAKE

- For heart failure: 2000-3000 mg./day; ideally less than 2000mg./day
- For everyone else: less than 2400 mg./day

REMEMBER...

1 teaspoon of salt contains 2000 mg. of sodium

Sodium guidelines

Our bodies don't require much sodium and most people can get enough without eating anything that tastes salty. Salt is only one of many substances that contain sodium. Other sodium sources are listed in the following table.

Since the taste for salt is learned, it can also be unlearned. You will lose your preference for salty foods after a while. So be patient. And in the meantime, make generous use of the other seasonings described later in this section.

If you have heart failure: choose most of your foods from the "LOW" column.
If you have high blood pressure: choose mostly from the "MODERATE" and "LOW" columns. Everyone else should eat mainly from the "MODERATE" and "LOW" columns, and limit high-sodium foods to a few times per week.

LOW **0-140 mg./serving**	**MODERATE** **140-300 mg./serving**	**HIGH** **300+ mg./serving**
Fresh meat, fish and poultry such as beef, pork, lamb, chicken, turkey, fish, seafood	Low-sodium canned chicken or tuna	Cured meats like ham, bacon, sausage Processed meats like hot dogs, luncheon meat, pre-basted turkey Frozen dinners or entrees, like fish sticks, burritos Canned tuna or salmon
Milk, yogurt Ice cream Cream cheese (1 Tbs.) Eggs	Natural cheeses (Swiss, cheddar, etc.) Buttermilk Egg substitute	Cottage cheese Processed cheese Cheese spreads
Fresh fruits and fruit juices Fresh vegetables Frozen vegetables (except peas, limas) Dried beans, peas and lentils	Frozen peas, limas Vegetables frozen in sauce Canned vegetables, drained and rinsed	Pickled foods including olives and sauerkraut Tomato juice or V8 Canned vegetables or beans Beans cooked with ham
Unsalted nuts, crackers, chips, pretzels Bread sticks Candy Jell-O Popsicles	Salted crackers Graham crackers French fries Popcorn Salted nuts (1 oz.) Donuts, cake, cookies	Salted chips, pretzels Cheese crackers Mincemeat pie
Bread, rolls Corn tortillas Pasta, potato or rice Hot cereal, oatmeal Shredded Wheat, puffed wheat or rice	Muffin or English muffin Biscuit Most cold cereals Scalloped, au gratin or mashed potatoes	Cornbread Pancakes, waffle Flour tortilla Instant oatmeal packets Rice, potatoes or stuffing from mix

| Canned tomato paste
Lemon juice
Herbs and spices
Herb Ox Very Low Sodium Instant Broth | Mustard and catsup
BBQ sauce (1 Tbsp.)
Salad dressing (1 Tbsp.) | Gravy or sauce from can, jar or mix (like Ragú)
Canned tomato sauce
Salt, "lite" salt, garlic salt, celery salt, etc.
Soy sauce, lite soy sauce |
| Unsalted peanut butter | Peanut butter
Low-salt Campbell's soup | Canned soup or broth
Dry soup mix |

Using less sodium in cooking

- Adapt your recipes by using half the amount of salt, or less. The Herbs and Spices chart later in this section will help you select other flavorings to use instead. Eventually, you will be able to leave out the salt completely.
- Change certain cooking techniques. For example, you don't need to add salt to water when cooking pasta, vegetables, rice or hot cereal.
- Replace salty condiments such as onion salt, celery salt, garlic salt, soy sauce and mustard. Use onion powder, garlic powder or other herbs and spices to enhance flavor.
- Use lemon juice instead of salt in salad dressings, fish and poultry dishes.
- Use homemade chicken broth for soups and gravies, or Very Low Sodium Instant Broth packets (made by Herb Ox.)

Using less sodium at the table

Remove the salt shaker from the table so you will be less tempted to add salt out of habit.

- If you still cannot shake the salt habit, consider switching the salt and pepper shakers. That is, put salt into the pepper shaker, which has fewer holes, so you use less.
- Avoid condiments that are high in sodium like catsup, soy sauce, mustard, steak sauce, and Worcestershire sauce. Some hot sauces (like La Victoria "Salsa Brava") contain little sodium and are OK to use in moderation. Check labels to be sure.
- Use pepper or herb blends (such as Mrs. Dash or Parsley Patch) instead of salt

Nutrition Facts
Serving Size 2/3 cup (55g)
Servings Per Container About 8

Amount Per Serving	
Calories 230	Calories from Fat 72
	% Daily Value*
Total Fat 8g	**12%**
Saturated Fat 1g	**5%**
Trans Fat 0g	
Cholesterol 0mg	**0%**
Sodium 160mg	**7%**
Total Carbohydrate 37g	**12%**
Dietary Fiber 4g	**16%**
Sugars 1g	
Protein 3g	
Vitamin A	10%
Vitamin C	8%
Calcium	20%
Iron	45%

* Percent Daily Values are based on a 2,000 calorie diet. Your daily value may be higher or lower depending on your calorie needs.

	Calories:	2,000	2,500
Total Fat	Less than	65g	80g
Sat Fat	Less than	20g	25g
Cholesterol	Less than	300mg	300mg
Sodium	Less than	2,400mg	2,400mg
Total Carbohydrate		300g	375g
Dietary Fiber		25g	30g

Nutrition Facts	
8 servings per container	
Serving size	**2/3 cup (55g)**

Amount per serving	
Calories	**230**
	% Daily Value*
Total Fat 8g	**10%**
Saturated Fat 1g	**5%**
Trans Fat 0g	
Cholesterol 0mg	**0%**
Sodium 160mg	**7%**
Total Carbohydrate 37g	**13%**
Dietary Fiber 4g	**14%**
Total Sugars 12g	
Includes 10g Added Sugars	**20%**
Protein 3g	
Vitamin D 2mcg	10%
Calcium 260mg	20%
Iron 8mg	45%
Potassium 235mg	6%

* The % Daily Value (DV) tells you how much a nutrient in a serving of food contributes to a daily diet. 2,000 calories a day is used for general nutrition advice.

Reading labels

It is very important that you, and anyone who buys food for you, can read product labels to find low-sodium foods. The new dietary food label is located below on the right. For those with heart failure the serving size[1], calories[2] and sodium amount[3] which is located in the middle of the label are key in reviewing food items.

Watch for these words on food labels and ingredient lists:

- Salt
- Sodium
- Baking soda
- Brine
- Monosodium glutamate

These words identify products that contain sodium. A general rule is to avoid all products that list salt or sodium among the first 5 ingredients on the label. A better rule is to read the "Nutrition Facts" label to find out how much sodium a product contains.

What to look for and avoid

The word "sodium" or "salt" among the first 5 ingredients.
Sodium content of 140 mg. or more per serving.

MINESTRONE SOUP RECIPE

This minestrone soup has been modified to be low in sodium. The list of ingredients may seem long, but they are mostly seasonings. Serve with crusty bread for a simple supper. Makes 6 generous servings.

Ingredients:

4 cups low-sodium broth or water
1 can (6 oz.) tomato paste or 4 tomatoes, coarsely chopped
1/3 cup uncooked barley
1 medium onion, chopped
1 potato, cut into 1" cubes
1/2 cup fresh parsley, chopped
2 bay leaves
2 tsp. dried basil
1 tsp. dried oregano
¼ tsp. each thyme, garlic powder
¼ tsp. black pepper or seasoned (spicy) pepper
2 ribs celery, cut into bite sized pieces
1-2 carrots, cut into bite sized pieces
1 cup cut-up vegetables (broccoli, cauliflower, zucchini, green beans, or a combination)
1 cup cooked beans (garbanzos, kidney, etc.)
½ cup uncooked macaroni

Instructions:

In a large pot, combine liquid with tomato paste or chopped tomatoes. Add barley, onion, potatoes, and seasonings, including parsley. Bring to a boil over medium heat, and simmer, covered, while you clean and cut the vegetables. Add chopped vegetables to the pot and simmer until vegetables are tender. Add cooked beans and macaroni, and simmer 10 minutes more, until macaroni is cooked.

Interpreting sodium labels

Food labels must show the sodium content of the food. You can compare the different brands of a particular food to find the one with the lowest sodium level. Try to choose products with no more than 140 mg. of sodium per serving. Labeling terms that can help you sort out the low-sodium and VERY low-sodium products are:

TERM	MEANING
Reduced salt	Usual sodium level reduced by 25% or more
Low sodium	140 mg of sodium or less per serving
Very low sodium	35 mg of sodium or less per serving
Sodium free	Less than 5 mg of sodium per serving
Unsalted (no added salt)	A normally salted food prepared without salt

Additional tips

At the Grocery Store:

- Buy fresh or frozen vegetables, since they are lower in sodium than canned.
- If you use canned vegetables, drain off the liquid and rinse the vegetables. Or look for brands with no added salt.
- Rinse canned tuna with tap water or choose low sodium or dietetic tuna fish.
- When buying frozen meals, choose the lowest levels of sodium possible. If you have heart failure, look for frozen meals with 500 mg of sodium or LESS for a complete meal.
- Beware of tomato products such as canned tomatoes and tomato sauce. Look for "no salt added" varieties. Tomato paste usually has no added sodium.
- Most canned soups are very high in sodium. Look for low sodium varieties that contain less than 140 mg. sodium per serving or make your own. (See recipe below) Even soups labeled "1/3 Less Sodium" contain too much at 580 mg/serving.

At the Restaurant:

- In restaurants, ask for dishes cooked without salt or high-sodium.
- flavorings like MSG. Order gravies, sauces and salad dressings on the side so you can add them sparingly.
- Beware of fast food. Nearly all their foods contain lots of sodium.

Herb blends

To reduce your use of salt, try different herb blends found in the supermarket. Some common commercial blends are Vegit, Mrs. Dash and Parsley Patch. Avoid the herb blends that contain salt

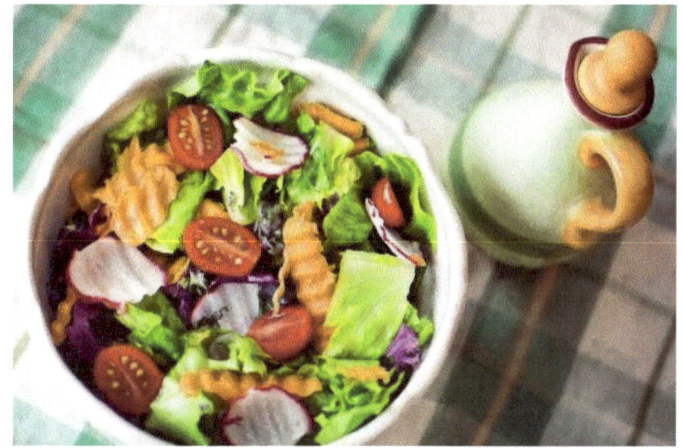

or are labeled low-sodium. These still contain too much sodium.

You can also try different seasonings when preparing food. Without salt, you may need to use more seasonings than usual so don't be timid. The herb and spice chart on the next page will help. Other seasonings that may be used in moderation include:

- Very Low Sodium Instant Broth (made by Herb Ox)
- Salsa Brava hot taco sauce (by La Victoria)
- Seasoned pepper (any brand that does not contain salt)

Salt substitutes

Most heart failure patients should avoid using salt substitutes (potassium chloride) because of the danger of potassium build-up in the body. If you have high blood pressure, you may try a salt substitute if you are sure you are not already taking potassium in some form. Check with your doctor or nurse before buying or using a salt substitute made with potassium.

Extra help for high blood pressure

Thanks to recent studies from the National Institutes of Health, we have learned more about preventing and treating high blood pressure. The DASH findings -- Dietary Approaches to Stop

Hypertension -- point to a diet that is naturally high in potassium, magnesium and calcium. These three minerals may help the body maintain a normal blood pressure. Foods containing these beneficial minerals include:

- Vegetables, especially dark green leafy ones
- Fruits and fruit juice
- Low-fat or fat-free dairy foods (milk, yogurt and cheese)
- Nuts, seeds, dried beans or lentils

Make a Plan

Now it's time to identify habits that you will try to change in the next week or two. Check the boxes for changes you will make. Put a star by items that you have already mastered. Keep working until you can put a star by every item.

- ☐ I will use sodium-free or very low sodium seasonings on my food instead of salt and salty condiments.
- ☐ I will read labels for sodium content and sodium-containing ingredients.
- ☐ When buying canned or packaged foods, I will try to choose ones with 140 mg. of sodium or less per serving.
- ☐ Every day I will eat two extra servings of fruit and vegetables, and at least two servings of low-fat or nonfat dairy foods.
- ☐ I will limit how often I eat cheese, cottage cheese or any food containing cheese.
- ☐ I will avoid pickled or salted snacks such olives, pickles, and salted chips, nuts, and pretzels.
- ☐ I will avoid eating salty or cured meats (ham, hot dogs, bacon, luncheon meats, etc.).
- ☐ Other ideas:

____

Low-sodium snacks

The best way to find low-sodium snacks is to choose fresh, unprocessed foods. If you choose packaged foods, read the labels to be sure the food is very low in sodium. Here are some guidelines for choosing low-sodium snacks:

- Read food labels for sodium content before buying or eating packaged foods.
- Choose foods with less than 100 mg of sodium per serving. Foods with 100-140 mg of sodium are okay if you don't have them every day.
- Compare different brands and choose the one with the least sodium.

More tips

- Make foods such as bread and bagels more interesting by adding a small amount (1 teaspoon) of margarine or cream cheese.
- Use jam, jelly and preserves, also. These contain almost no sodium.
- Snack on leftovers: homemade soup, vegetables, potatoes, etc.

The snack foods suggested here contain less than 140 mg of sodium. Pay attention to serving sizes; some are rather small.

FOOD	Amount	FOOD	Amount
Angel cake*	1 slice	Gingersnaps*	2-3
Applesauce*	½ cup	Graham crackers	2 sq.
Bagel	1	Jell-O*	½ cup
Bread or toast	1-2 sl	Marshmallows*	2-3
Breadsticks (unsalted)	2	Nuts (unsalted)	¼ cup
Candy*(gum drops, hard candies, jelly beans)	several	Popcorn (unsalted)	3 cups
		Popsicle, fudge bar*	1
Corn tortilla	1-2	Pretzels (unsalted)	½ cup
Crackers (unsalted)	3-5	Puffed wheat/rice cereal	1 cup
Dried fruit*(raisins, etc.)	¼ cup	Unsalted Rice cakes	2
Fresh fruit*	1-2	Sherbet*	½ -1 cup
Fruit juice* (not tomato)	½ cup	Shredded wheat cereal	1 cup
Fig bars*	2-3	Vanilla wafers*	3-5
Low-fat frozen desserts*	½ -1 cup	Yogurt*(read labels)	1 cup

*Diabetic patients should limit fruit & sweets. Choose foods without a star.

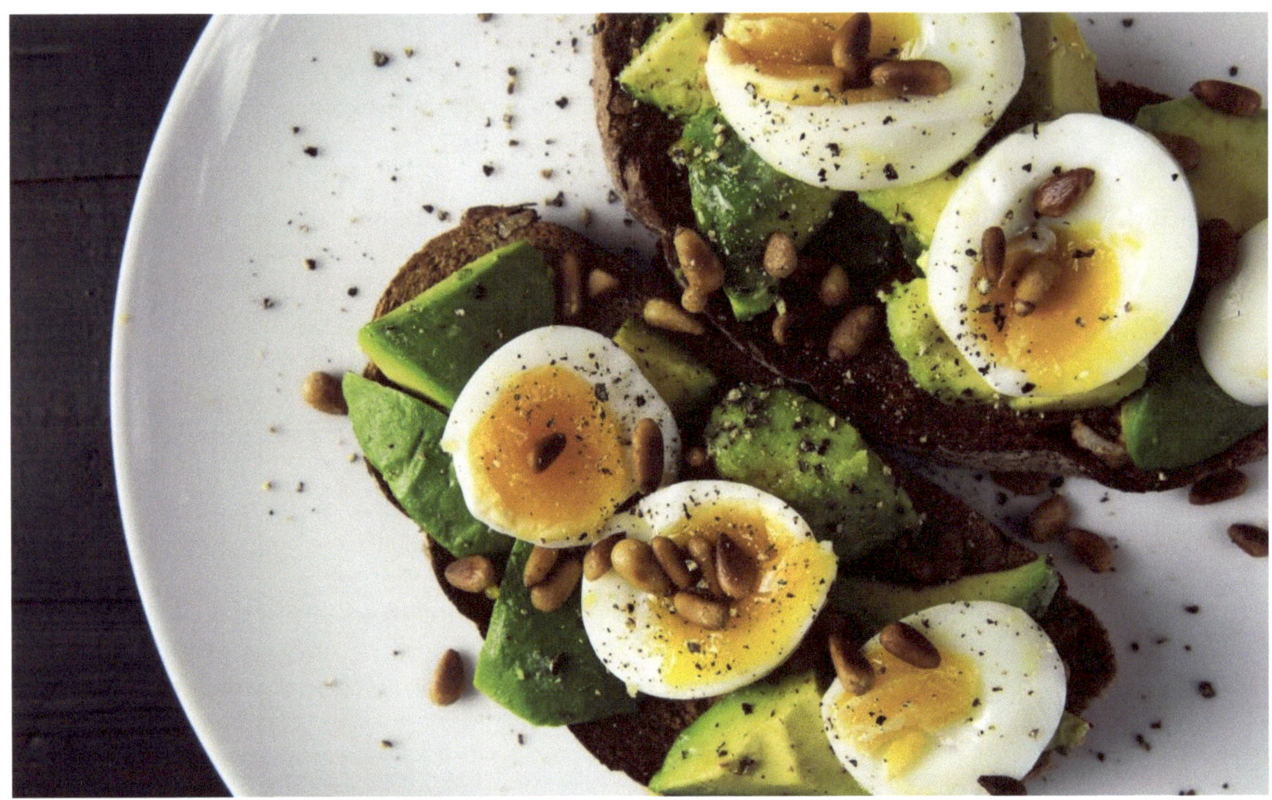

EATING AWAY FROM HOME

People with heart failure are usually able to eat out and enjoy social eating with friends and family. However, you must be careful to select low-sodium foods no matter where you eat. Here are some suggestions to help you eat away from home on a low-sodium diet.

In general

- Eat something before you leave home, so won't be so hungry that you make poor choices when you're out.
- If you drink alcohol, limit yourself to one drink. It's better for your heart and your willpower.
- Look for "sure bets", such as fresh fruit, raw vegetables and bread. Be cautious about everything else.
- Take along some low-sodium food or snacks, just In case.
- Ask questions about what's in a food and how it was prepared.

- Be extra strict about sodium the rest of the day, since you are likely to have more sodium than usual whenever you eat away from home.

At restaurants

- Explain to your waiter that you cannot eat salt and ask that he/she help you select a salt-free meal. (Talk about "salt" rather than "sodium", to be sure the waiter understands.)
- Choose plain, simply prepared foods as much as possible. Select items such as:
  - broiled or roasted meat, chicken or fish
  - baked potato with toppings on the side (so you can add just a little)
  - salad, without dressing, or add oil and vinegar/lemon juice yourself

- fresh vegetables, cooked to order without salt
- sherbet or fresh fruit for dessert
- Bring along a salt-free salad dressing and herb blend to sprinkle on your meal.

At the homes of friends and relatives

- Let your hosts know that you must follow a very strict diet. Assure them that you are happy for the invitation even if you may not be able to eat.
- If you are very comfortable with your hosts, ask them to prepare a dish or two without salt, canned foods, or other high-sodium ingredients.
- Offer to bring a dish to contribute to the meal, so you can be sure of having at least one thing you can eat safely.

At parties and social events

- If appropriate, use the tips for eating with friends and relatives (above).
- Stay far from where the food is located, so you won't be tempted to nibble.
- Sip a glass of water or a soft drink so you have something in your hands.
- Focus on other aspects of the event: dancing, talking, meeting people. There are lots of ways to be social without eating and drinking.

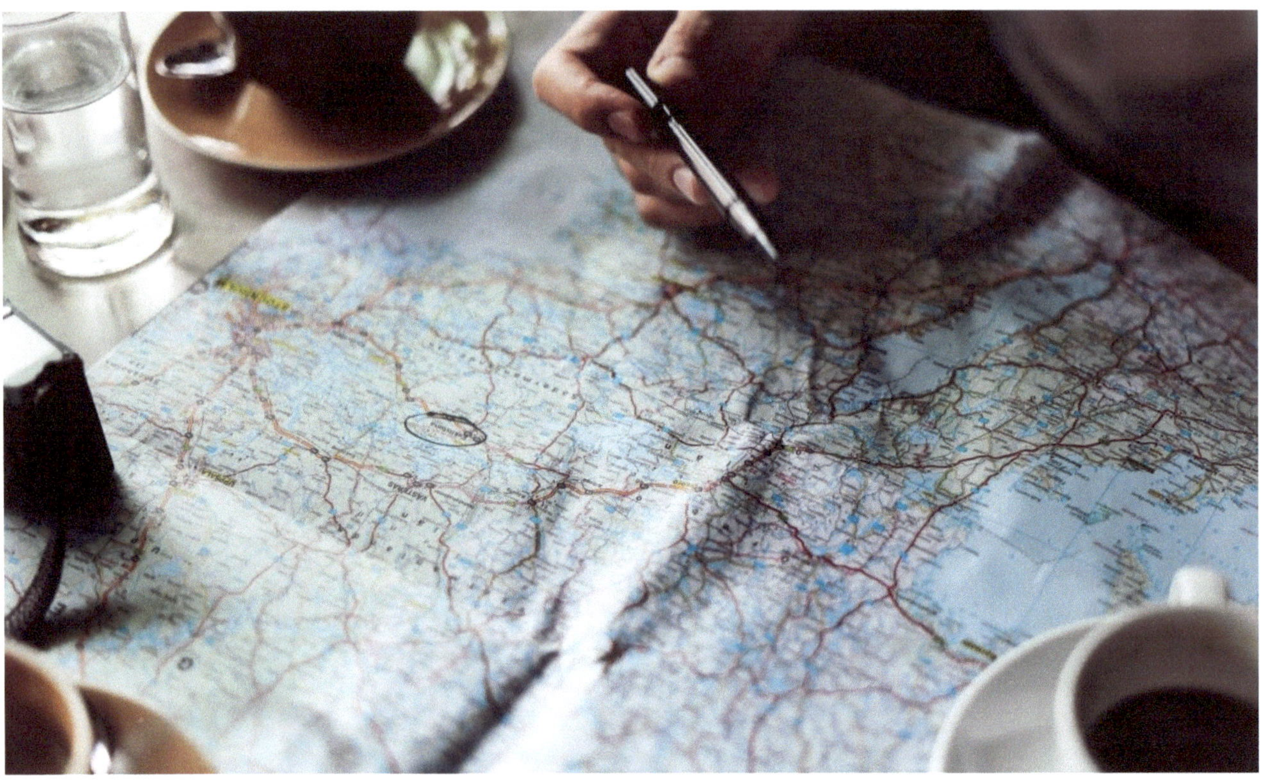

VACATION AND TRAVEL TIPS

Advance planning can help you have a safe, relaxing trip whenever you travel. Here are some guidelines to help you prepare for vacations and other trips:

Talk with your doctor or nurse

- Discuss your travel plans: where you're going, when, and what you plan to do.
- Obtain a referral for a doctor and hospital at each place you'll visit, just in case you might need them.
- Ask for a summary of your medical condition and a copy of your E.K.G. (electrocardiogram) to take with you.
- Keep a list of your medicines with you.

Talk to your agent or airline

- Avoid travel to places that are very hot or very cold.

- Learn how much activity is required for a tour, or simply for getting around.
- Ask about wheelchair access, if necessary, and luggage handling.
- Request an aisle seat on airplanes so you can easily walk around or get to the restroom.
- Request special meals (low-sodium, low fat, diabetic if necessary) on the airplane.
- Request hotels with non-smoking rooms and a place to exercise.
- Ask for referrals to heart-healthy restaurants.

Plan Ahead

- Stop your mail and make other arrangements well before you leave. (You do not need to clean the whole house before you leave.)

- Start packing a week before you leave; use a checklist to help you remember everything.
- BRING YOUR SCALE if possible, to record your weights.
- Bring some snacks and other food in case you have trouble finding low-sodium foods.

While you're away

- Carry your medicines in your carry-on bag, not in your checked luggage.
- Always have someone help you with your luggage.
- Walk around and do ankle exercises on the airplane or bus. If you travel by car, stop every 1 to 2 hours to stretch your legs.
- Rest for the first 24 hours after you arrive, especially when traveling to other countries or to higher elevations.
- Call ahead to restaurants to be sure they prepare low-sodium foods.
- Stick with plain, simple foods when ordering meals. Avoid buffets and salad bars, where food may be salted.
- Avoid alcohol.
- Allow yourself time to rest during the day.
- Plan to skip one activity or side trip every day so you have time to rest up for your next event.
- Avoid activity right after you eat.
- Dress for the weather.
- Have a wonderful, relaxing time.

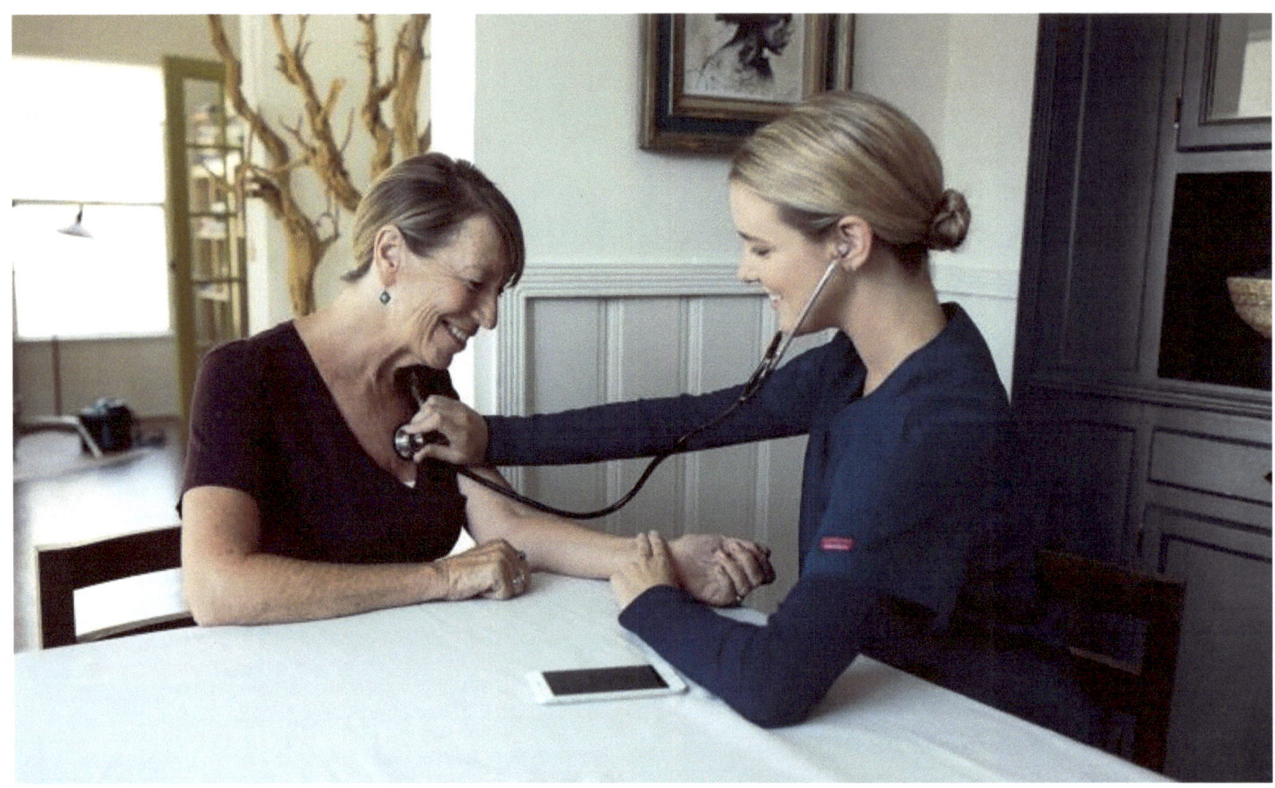

COMMUNICATING WITH YOUR DOCTOR

It is important to get the most out of your visits with your doctor. There can be a lot of information to remember and some can be forgotten as soon as you leave. Preparing for your visits can help you to understand and communicate your needs more effectively.

Take the quiz below to see how you are doing:

- ☐ I always write down my questions before I go to a visit with my doctor.
- ☐ I take notes during my visit or record instructions on my phone or tape recorder.
- ☐ I speak up and tell my doctor when I'm not sure about his/her instructions.
- ☐ I always bring a list of my current medicines to my visit.
- ☐ I can repeat back all the instructions my doctor gave me before I leave his office.

- ☐ I ask my doctor to write down all the things I need to know when I get home.

If you responded "no' to any of these, follow these tips to get more out of your doctor visits:

Tip #1
Don't be afraid to speak up! Be sure to raise concerns you may have about taking a medicine, weighing yourself daily, or symptoms that are causing you worry. There are no dumb questions and it is better to know more, than less.

Tip #2
Clarify what you hear. There will be a lot of information to take in, and you want to be sure that you understand what the doctor is telling you. Ask your doctor to repeat special instructions and explain terminology that you are unfamiliar with.

You may want to try repeating what you've heard, it can help you to commit it to memory. Write special instructions down in case you need to reference them later.

Tip #3
Prepare for every visit. Doctors and nurses can provide better care if they know what you need from a visit. Prepare an up-to- date list of all of the medicines you are taking (including over-the-counter) and a list any symptoms you are having. Be sure to ask about treatments or medicines that may help with those symptoms and tests, procedures and follow-up appointments. Think about asking a family member to write down important instructions the doctor gives you during a visit and don't hesitate to call or email your doctor if you forget or are unclear on those instructions.

Remember: Better communication leads to better care.

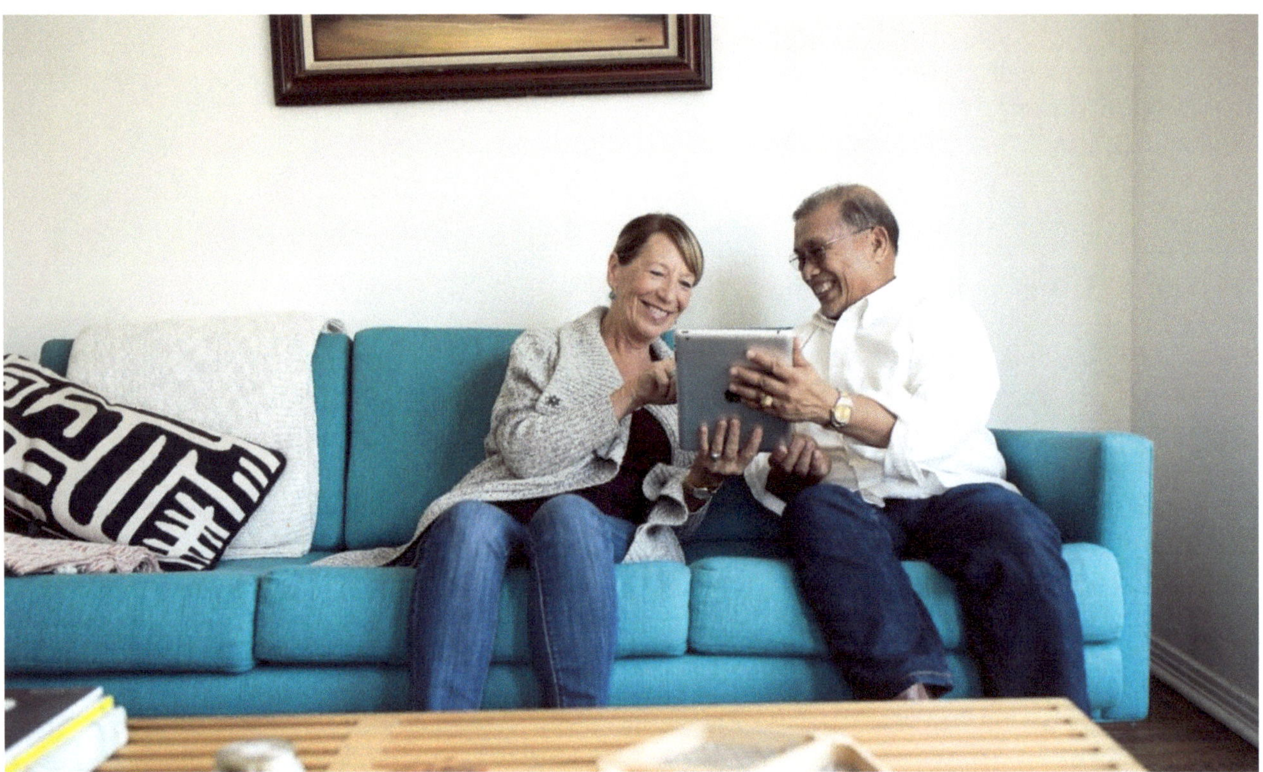

INFORMATION FOR FAMILY AND FRIENDS

You can help your relative or friend take care of his/her heart failure in two ways: (1) learn about the disease and its treatment, and (2) ask him/her to make the lifestyle changes that help to control the symptoms.

Take Care of Yourself

- Don't be afraid to ask questions of all health care professionals, especially the doctor. You need to know what's going on.
- Reduce stress at home. Set aside time for you and your relative or friend to talk or sit together quietly. Talk about your concerns and needs.
- Remember that you are not in charge of his/her health. He/she needs to take responsibility for their health.

Help with Medicines

- Ask your relative or friend how you can help them remember to take their medicines.

- Help them remember to have the doctor renew their prescriptions a week before they run out. He/she should call the pharmacy for medicine refills 5-7 days in advance.

Know About Symptom Changes

- Post the doctor's telephone number(s) at home. Talk with other household members about calling for help if symptoms occur.
- Know the warning signs that heart failure is getting worse. Encourage your relative or friend to report new or worsening symptoms right away, including weight gain.

Help with Diet Changes

- Take a shopping trip to the grocery store together. Read labels and select foods that appeal to both of you and are low in sodium.

NOTES

NOTES

NOTES

NOTES

www.ingramcontent.com/pod-product-compliance
Lightning Source LLC
Chambersburg PA
CBHW040052240726
48664CB00004B/1163